THE
PERFECT

THREESOME

YOUR LONGEVITY BLUEPRINT

AUTHORED BY
TORY TREWHITT

Paperback ISBN:	**978-1-923650-05-3**
Author:	**Tory Trewhitt**
Editor:	**Lynette Reurts**
Cover Graphics:	**Mylen Carascal**

A catalogue record for this book is available from the National Library
of Australia.

DISCLAIMER
The information contained in this book is for general informational
purposes only. The author and publisher are not offering any medical,
legal or professional advice. While every effort has been made to ensure
the accuracy and completeness of the information provided, the author
and publisher assume no responsibility for errors or omissions or any
outcomes or consequences resulting from using this book's content.

COPYRIGHT
All original material in this book is the sole property of the author and
Morpheus Publishing.

DISTRIBUTION
This book is distributed by Morpheus Publishing and is available
through authorised distributors, booksellers, Morpheus Publishing
website.

COPYRIGHT PERMISSIONS
For copyright permissions or any other inquiries, please contact:

PUBLISHER: Morpheus Publishing
www.morpheuspublishing.com.au || hello@justinemartin.com.au ||
+61403 564 942

AUTHOR: Tory Trewhitt
https://www.morpheuspublishing.com.au/authors/tory-trewhitt

TABLE OF CONTENTS

INTRODUCTION

"Life is a game, you make the rules."

~ Tory Trewhitt

Tory Trewhitt is a powerhouse in the world of health and human performance. An Exercise Physiologist, Accountability Coach, Motivational Speaker, Trainer, and Author, he has spent decades educating, motivating, and inspiring others to take charge of their health and lifestyle. His passion has always been simple, but powerful: *helping one to help many.*

Through his unique ability to connect, simplify, and empower, Tory has guided countless people toward living with more energy, purpose, and balance. He believes health isn't about perfection; it's about progress, structure, and consistency. His mission is to help individuals, families, and workplaces build sustainable habits that create lasting change. After all, life is for living.

Following the success of his first book, *Blokes Inc. Play a Bigger Game*, Tory realised that, while the message resonated deeply with men, there was a whole community of women, families, and younger generations who also needed a framework for sustainable wellness. So, *The Perfect Threesome* was born.

This quick, easy-read *'wellness blueprint'* simplifies the foundations of health into three essential pillars: **Sleep, Nutrition, and Exercise**, supported by **Emotional Wellness** and **Social Connectivity.** It's designed to give you the clarity, motivation, and structure to kickstart your own wellness journey and live a life full of vitality. Each chapter in the book follows a clear, practical format, delivering three key insights on the topics and three simple, actionable steps the reader must implement as part of their daily ritual, ensuring real progress, real habits, and real change.

Knowing Tory, this is only the beginning. *CHICKS INC.* and *KIDS INC.* may not be far behind, because his mission extends beyond individuals to creating healthier, happier communities.

We trust you'll enjoy this read and, more importantly, share it with those you care about. Here's to improving your *Perfect Threesome* and playing a bigger game with your health and your life.

CHAPTER 1

SLEEP:
The Forgotten Superpower

"If you're not sleeping, you're not recovering. If you're not recovering, you're not growing."

~ Tory Trewhitt

L et's get this straight from the start: sleep isn't a luxury, it's a non-negotiable. You can train hard in the gym, eat clean, and hustle hard, but if your sleep is rubbish, you're running on empty. Think of sleep as your body's natural performance enhancer. It's where your muscles rebuild, your mind resets, and your hormones find balance. Without it, everything else, your mood, focus, relationships, and your energy starts to crumble.

When you sleep, your body's doing more than just resting. It's running a full overnight service. Your heart rate slows, your breathing steadies, and your body shifts into repair mode. Growth hormone is released to rebuild muscle tissue. Your immune system recharges. Your brain clears out mental clutter and locks in memories from the day. A study referenced by the National Institute of Health (NIH) found that consistent quality sleep supports the production and priming of key immune system cells, the building blocks of our innate immunity.

Miss out on that, and the impact is brutal:

- You feel flat and foggy.

- Your reaction time slows.

- You crave sugar and carbs.
- Your motivation tanks.

Here's the kicker: long-term sleep deprivation raises your risk of heart disease, diabetes, depression, and even weight gain. So, when you tell yourself you'll "catch up later," you're kidding yourself. You can't out-train, out-eat, or out-hustle poor sleep habits.

Sleep is the base layer of your performance pyramid. Without quality, consistent sleep, the whole thing collapses.

THE MYTHS WE STILL BELIEVE

Let's bust a few big ones.

Myth #1: "I only need five hours, I'm fine."

Nah, you're not. You've just normalised exhaustion. Chronic sleep debt tricks your brain into thinking this half-alive version of you is your best, but it's not.

Myth #2: "I'll sleep when I'm dead."

You'll just get there quicker. Lack of sleep is linked to everything from heart issues to burnout.

Myth #3: "A little drink will help me sleep."

Alcohol might knock you out, but it destroys your sleep quality. You'll wake up dehydrated, restless, and far from recovered.

The truth is simple: high performers don't brag about surviving on less, they actually protect their sleep like a secret weapon. Change your mindset = change your performance and change your sleeping habits.

SIMPLE STRATEGIES FOR BETTER SLEEP

Sleep doesn't just happen, it's a skill, and like any skill, it takes practice and consistency. Here's how to start sleeping like a pro:

1. Create a wind-down routine.

An hour before bed, start powering down. Dim the lights, stretch, breathe, or read something that doesn't fire up your brain. Your body needs signals that it's time to switch off.

2. Make your bedroom a sleep zone.

Dark, cool, and quiet that's the formula. Get rid of the clutter, lower the temperature to around 18°C, and invest in a good mattress and pillows.

3. Cut the tech.

Your phone is the enemy of deep sleep. Blue light messes with melatonin (your sleep hormone), and late-night scrolling keeps your mind wired. Set a phone curfew, no screens 30 – 60 minutes before bed.

4. Keep it consistent.

Go to bed and wake up at the same time, even on the weekends. Your body loves rhythm, and consistency builds better quality sleep.

5. Watch your caffeine and alcohol.

Caffeine has a six-hour half-life, meaning that the coffee you drank at 3 p.m. could still be keeping you up at 9. So that 'nightcap' might make you drowsy, but it'll wreck your Rapid Eye Movement (REM) sleep. REM is the restorative sleep stage where your brain becomes highly active, dreams occur, and important processes like emotional regulation, memory consolidation and learning takes place.

THE 'SLEEP LIKE IT'S YOUR JOB' MINDSET

Here's the shift: stop treating sleep as downtime and start treating it as your next-day performance prep. Change your mindset to being an athlete and then ask yourself: do athletes pull all-nighters before competition? CEOs at the top of their game don't boast about fatigue, so neither should you. When you prioritise sleep, everything else levels up. Your energy, focus, strength, patience, libido, and confidence. It's the edge most of us overlook. So, make it part of your daily non-negotiables. Protect your sleep window. Plan your nights like you plan your workouts. Don't just go to bed, recover like a professional.

Remember, sleep isn't lazy. It's leadership. It's showing up for your body, your brain, and your family at full capacity. So, tonight, skip the late-night Netflix, power down early, and make your bedroom your recovery zone, because every hour of quality sleep is an investment.

TOP 3 TIPS TO IMPROVE YOUR SLEEP

1. SET A CONSISTENT ROUTINE

Go to bed and wake up at the same time every day — even on weekends.
This anchors your body's internal clock, improving sleep quality and energy levels.

2. CREATE A SLEEP SANCTUARY

Keep your bedroom cool, dark, and quiet.
Remove screens, dim the lights an hour before bed, and invest in a comfortable mattress and pillow.

3. WIND DOWN, DON'T POWER DOWN

Build a pre-sleep ritual stretch, read, meditate, or journal.
Avoid caffeine, alcohol, and screens 1—2 hours before bed to help your body naturally shift into rest mode.

LIST THREE ACTIONABLE STEPS TO IMPROVE YOUR SLEEP

1._____

2._____

3._____

CHAPTER 2

NUTRITION:
Fuel, Don't Fill

"When diet is wrong, medicine is of no use. When diet is correct, medicine is of no need."

~ Ayurvedic proverb

When it comes to food, most of us eat for comfort, not for performance. We eat because we're stressed, bored, or celebrating. The problem? Those moments add up, and before you know it, you're tired, bloated, and wondering why your energy's gone missing.

Nutrition isn't about dieting or deprivation, it's about fuelling your body to perform. Food is your most powerful tool for energy, focus, recovery, and longevity. Get it right, and everything else, training, sleep, mood falls into place.

FOOD AS ENERGY VS. FOOD AS COMFORT

Here's the truth: food should serve you, not soothe you.

Yes, it's okay to enjoy your meals, but it's not okay to rely on them to manage stress, boredom, or emotion. That's where most of us trip up. When you shift your mindset from comfort to fuel, everything changes.

You start asking better questions:

   ● You Will this give me energy or take it away?

- Will this help me recover or slow me down?

- Will I feel better or worse an hour after eating it?

THE HONESTY TRAPS (THREESOME): BOOZE, SUGAR, AND PROCESSED RUBBISH

Let's call it how it is: most of us fall into the same three traps.

1. Booze

Alcohol is social, cultural, and often part of winding down, but it's also a recovery killer. It slows muscle repair, messes with hormones, dehydrates you, and ruins sleep. You don't need to quit completely, you just need to be smart. Save it for weekends, occasions, or celebrations. You'll enjoy it more and feel sharper for it.

2. Sugar

Sugar is sneaky. It's in sauces, cereals, snacks, and 'healthy' drinks. It spikes your blood sugar, crashes your energy, and drives cravings. Learn to read labels and remember, if sugar's in the top three ingredients, leave it on the shelf.

3. Processed rubbish

If it comes in a box, bag, or packet and lasts longer than your home loan, it's probably not serving you. Stick to real food and seasonal eating. Keep it basic: meat, fish, eggs, fruit, vegetables, nuts, and whole grains. Real food doesn't need marketing, it just needs making.

BUILDING A SUSTAINABLE PLATE: PROTEIN, PLANTS, HEALTHY FATS, AND BALANCE

Forget complicated diets, just keep it simple. Every plate should have four things:

1. Protein – The building block for muscle and recovery. Aim to include lean sources like chicken, fish, eggs, or plant-based proteins with every meal.

2. Plants – Eat the rainbow. Different colours equal different nutrients. Veggies fuel your gut, boost immunity, and keep inflammation down.

3. Healthy Fats – Avocado, olive oil, nuts, seeds, and oily fish. They support brain health, hormones, and joint function.

4. Balance – You don't need to be perfect. You just need to be consistent. The key is portion control, not overeating even the good stuff as all food contains calories.

Think: real food, right portions, regular timing.

Remember, perfection isn't sustainable, and neither is guilt. The 80/20 rule is the sweet spot: eat clean 80% of the time and enjoy yourself the other 20%. Have the pizza. Drink the beer or have that glass of wine with a little dessert. Just don't let it become your default. The goal is control, not restriction. When you're consistent most of the time, your body forgives the rest. Food is meant to add to your life, not dominate it.

It's simple: when you fuel properly, you think clearer, move better, and feel unstoppable. Nutrition isn't a short-term project, it needs to become a lifelong partnership with your body. Every meal is a chance to feel better, perform stronger, and recover faster. So, next time you reach for a snack or pour a drink, ask yourself: *Am I fuelling my body or just filling it?*

The key is choosing fuel: choose energy and choose longevity. That's how you build a body and a life that performs for decades.

TOP 3 TIPS TO IMPROVE YOUR NUTRITION

1. EAT REAL, WHOLE FOODS

Build your meals around fresh, minimally processed ingredients, lean proteins, colourful vegetables, whole grains, and healthy fats. Real food fuels real energy.

2. BALANCE YOUR PLATE

Aim for a **simple ½—¼—¼ rule:**

- ½ plate veggies or salad
- ¼ lean protein
- ¼ complex carbs.

Add a drizzle of healthy fat for flavour and satiety.

3. MASTER CONSISTENCY, NOT PERFECTION

Nourishment comes from habits, not quick fixes. Stay hydrated, plan ahead, and focus on progress over perfection. Small daily improvements create long-term change.

LIST THREE ACTIONABLE STEPS TO IMPROVE YOUR NUTRITION

1._____

2._____

3._____

CHAPTER 3

EXERCISE:
Move with Purpose

"Exercise isn't about punishment or perfection, it's a daily reminder that you're built to move, built to grow, and built to handle whatever life throws at you."

~ Tory Trewhitt

When it comes to living like a high-performer, movement is the great equaliser. Exercise isn't punishment for what you ate, it's a celebration of what your body can do. Whether you're lifting weights, hiking a mountain, or chasing your kids around the backyard, movement fuels confidence, sharpens focus, and builds resilience from the inside out. Yet too many of us don't do it or respect it. Exercise is the 3rd Pillar to Optimal Wellbeing, and in this chapter, you will discover why movement matters, not just for vanity, but for vitality as well. Personally, I think is it the primary pillar for optimising your health and wellbeing, both physically and emotionally.

MOVEMENT AS MEDICINE

You have heard it before, that movement is medicine. We know that exercise is the closest thing we have to a miracle drug, and the best part is, it's free. Regular movement lowers your risk of chronic disease, boosts mood, improves sleep, and sharpens your thinking. It's a natural antidepressant, stress reliever, and energy booster all in one. If these effects were listed on a packet, in a potion or in a pill, you would take it every day, yet too many people don't exercise at all, and wonder why they function so poorly.

Beyond the science, movement reconnects you to yourself. It reminds you that you're capable of doing hard things. When you push through that last rep, up the last incline or hill, or complete that set, you're not just building muscle, you're training your mind to persist when life gets tough. The facts are simple: the best workout is the one you'll actually do consistently. Forget chasing trends, I have written about Bio-Hacking too many times. The key to success is to just do the basics well first and worry about bio-hacking later. Nevertheless, whatever you choose as your form of movement (weights, Pilates, Yoga, cycling, swimming etc), it must be something you enjoy so it is sustainable and you can stay committed to it.

PERFORMANCE, NOT PERFECTION

Unfortunately, too many people fall into the all-or-nothing trap. They go hard for six weeks, then life gets busy, and suddenly the gym shoes are gathering dust. Real progress isn't made in heroic bursts, it's built on small, consistent actions over time.

Train for performance, not perfection. That means focusing on becoming *better*, not chasing some unrealistic ideal. Maybe that's lifting a little heavier, running a little further, or recovering a little faster. The wins compound, physically and mentally.

When you view exercise as performance training for life, not punishment, everything changes. You stop asking, "How do I look?" and start asking, "How do I feel? How do I perform?"

However, it is not just about the cardiovascular (huff and puff); everyone needs a base of strength, and I talk a lot about the importance of eating protein and strength training (lifting heavy things) when I'm educating, inspiring and motivating people around 'optimal wellbeing'. Not just for muscle (skeletal strength), but for metabolism, posture, and confidence. Strength training teaches discipline, improves hormonal health, and helps protect your body from injury. It doesn't have to be complicated, it just needs to be consistent. Focus on the big movements that carry over to real life: squats, deadlifts, pushes, pulls, and carries. Train your body to lift, move, and perform. Yes, lift heavy things. It's good for your bones, hormone regulation, and your mindset, regardless of your age or gender. It's not about spending hours in the gym to stay active. The best bodies and minds are built by simply moving more throughout the day.

- Take the stairs.
- Walk after meals.
- Stretch while watching TV.
- Get outside every day: sunlight, fresh air, and movement are a potent combo.

Change your mindset to focus on non-exercise movement. Every step counts. Movement should be woven into the fabric of your life, not just something you schedule when you have time. The simple facts are if you don't move more, you'll eventually run out of time, not because the clock stops, but because your body does. When you don't exercise, you increase your risk of getting sick, losing your vitality and potentially cutting your life short.

RECOVERY IS PART OF THE PLAN

We all like a little downtime, and we need to start respecting that the 'rest' is where the magic happens.

Muscles don't grow during your workout, they grow during recovery. That means quality sleep, proper nutrition, hydration, and active rest days are just as important as the training itself. If you're constantly sore, exhausted, or irritable, you're not training smarter, you're burning out. The key to longevity is balancing intensity and training frequency with rest. Listen to your body. A rested human is a stronger human.

So it's time to change your mindset and respect that exercise isn't optional, it's actually a cornerstone of performance. Treat it like a non-negotiable meeting with yourself, because that's exactly what it is.

When you move with purpose, you're not just training your body, you're investing in your energy, focus, and emotional strength. You're teaching yourself discipline, resilience, and the ability to show up even when you don't feel like it. Every rep, run, ride, or stretch is a deposit into your longevity account. Move like it's your job because your health is your work. Exercise isn't just about aesthetics, it's about creating a body that supports the life you want to live. The stronger and fitter you become, the more capable, confident, and present you are for your work, your friends, and your family. When you move with purpose, you're not just playing the game, you're playing a bigger one.

TOP 3 TIPS TO IMPROVE YOUR EXERCISE HABITS

1. FIND YOUR WHY

Anchor your training to a meaningful purpose, such as energy for your kids, confidence in your body, or long-term health. A strong 'why' turns discipline into desire.

2. BUILD CONSISTENCY, NOT INTENSITY

Focus on showing up, not smashing every session. Start small, i.e. 20 minutes daily beats one big workout a week. Momentum creates motivation.

3. ADD ACCOUNTABILITY AND ENJOYMENT

Exercise with a friend, join a class, or hire a coach. Enjoyment and connection make habits stick and we know that when it is fun, it's for life.

LIST THREE ACTIONABLE STEPS TO IMPROVE YOUR EXERCISE ROUTINE

1._____

2._____

3._____

CHAPTER 4

STRESS:
Tame the Beast

"Not all stress is bad. The right kind of stress sharpens you, strengthens you, and reminds you that growth only happens when you step outside your comfort zone."

~ Tory Trewhitt

You can eat well, train hard, and sleep like a champion, but if you don't manage your stress, it will quietly dismantle everything you've built. Stress is the glue that holds life together when balanced and the acid that eats away at your health, energy, and mindset when it's not. Let's be honest: none of us are immune to stress. Work deadlines, financial pressure, relationships, family; it all piles up. The goal isn't to eliminate stress (you can't), but to *tame the beast* before it takes control of you.

Stress, in the right dose, is actually good for you. It sharpens focus, boosts performance, and drives adaptation. That's why a tough workout or a challenging project can leave you feeling alive and accomplished. The problem is when stress becomes chronic. When your nervous system never switches off, when your heart rate is always elevated, when your sleep is disrupted, and your mood is short fused. You are no longer growing; you are grinding yourself down. The key is to think of stress like fire: ideally small and controlled to keep you warm, not out of control so it burns everything in its path.

SIGNS YOU'RE RUNNING ON EMPTY

Unfortunately, most of us don't realise that we are stressed until something snaps: an argument, an illness, or complete burnout. So here are a few signs you might be tipping over the edge:

- You wake up tired, even after a full night's sleep.

- You crave sugar, caffeine, or alcohol just to get through the day.

- You've lost motivation to train, connect, or do what you enjoy.

- You're short-tempered, distracted, or constantly in 'fight or flight' mode.

Sound familiar? That's your body waving the white flag. It's time to recalibrate.

TOOLS TO TAME THE BEAST

1. Breathe — the reset button

Breathwork is one of the simplest and most powerful tools to calm your nervous system. Try a little box breathing: inhale deeply for 4 seconds, hold for 2, exhale slowly for 6. Repeat for a few minutes. It's a circuit breaker that brings you back to the present moment and out of your head.

2. Get outside — nature is medicine

There's something primal about fresh air, sunlight, and space. Nature doesn't judge, doesn't rush, and doesn't care about your inbox. Whether it's a surf, a bushwalk, or just sitting under a tree, being in nature helps lower cortisol, reduce anxiety, and restore perspective.

3. Write it out — empty the tank

Journaling isn't soft, it's smart — it's the performance edge. Getting your thoughts out of your head and onto paper helps you process what's weighing you down. You don't need to write poetry, just dump on the page whatever's on your mind, what you're grateful for, or what you want to change. It's therapy without the waiting room.

4. Unplug — reclaim your attention

Constant notifications, emails, and doom-scrolling keep your nervous system wired so start by setting boundaries. No phone at dinner. A digital sunset an hour before bed. Take weekends or evenings where you disconnect completely. Your mind needs downtime to recharge not just your body, but also your mind. Put the 'OUT OF OFFICE' response on your email, guilt free.

5. Move — the stress release valve

Exercise isn't just about muscle, it's about mindset. When you move your body, you release built-up tension and reset your brain chemistry. Whether it's lifting, running, or stretching, use movement as a release, not an obligation.

BUILDING STRESS RESILIENCE

Managing stress isn't about eliminating the load; it's about strengthening your frame. The more you build your foundation through The Perfect Threesome formula; sleep, nutrition, and movement, the better equipped you are to handle life's curveballs.

Think of stress like weight training: over time, you get stronger, not because the weight gets lighter, but because you do. That's what resilience really means: not avoiding hard things, but facing them with calm, control, and confidence.

Remember, there is a difference between working hard and burning out. If you're constantly exhausted, disconnected, or losing joy in the things you love, it's time to pause. Talk to someone: a friend, a coach, or a professional. I often ask people, 'who is on your TEAM?', because asking for help isn't weakness, it's wisdom. You don't need a big team, you just need a team. You can't pour from an empty cup, and the people who rely on you, family, colleagues, friends need you at your best, not at your breaking point.

It's important to note that stress will always be part of life, but how you respond defines the quality of it. Don't try to outmuscle stress; outsmart it. Build rituals that reset your body and mind daily. Breathe. Move. Rest. Reflect. Disconnect.

When you manage your stress, everything else, your energy, relationships, and performance falls into place. Once you respect stress, you'll find a calmer, stronger, more capable version of yourself waiting on the other side.

TOP 3 TIPS TO DECREASE STRESS

1. BREATHE AND BE PRESENT

Slow, deep breathing activates your parasympathetic nervous system, lowering heart rate and calming the mind. Try 4 — 6 slow breaths before meetings, workouts, or sleep.

2. MOVE YOUR BODY DAILY

Exercise releases endorphins, which are your body's natural stress relievers. Even a 10-minute walk, stretch, or swim can shift your mood and energy instantly.

3. CONNECT AND UNPLUG

Share your thoughts with a friend, partner, or colleague, because human connection soothes stress. Balance your digital life: less scrolling, more living.

LIST THREE ACTIONABLE STEPS TO IMPROVE YOUR STRESS LEVELS

1._____

2._____

3._____

CHAPTER 5

EMOTIONAL WELLNESS:
The Tough Stuff

"Real strength isn't about holding it all together: it's having the courage to open up, let go, and rebuild stronger than before."

~ Tory Trewhitt

L et's face it, emotional wellbeing is a key ingredient to longevity. Yet many of us aren't always great at talking about what's going on upstairs, particularly males. We're taught to toughen up, push through, and get on with it. But the truth is, real toughness isn't about bottling things up, it's about facing them head-on. This chapter is about emotional wellness and the inner game, because it doesn't matter how fit, how strong, or how successful you are on the outside if your mental game is falling apart on the inside.

For generations, many of us have been told that showing emotion equals weakness. But here's the twist: ignoring what's going on in your head doesn't make you strong, it makes you silent, and silence is where struggle grows.

The world is changing, and thankfully, so is the conversation. We're seeing more people open up about anxiety, depression, burnout, and stress, not as victims, but as humans. There's no shame in saying, *"I'm not okay right now."* Talking about mental health isn't soft. It's smart. It's courageous, and it's one of the best ways to protect yourself from reaching breaking point. Resilience isn't about pretending everything's fine, it's about learning how to bend without breaking. It's the skill of staying grounded when life hits you hard, and this is where mindset plays a huge role. Every setback, challenge, or mistake can be a teacher if you let it. Reflect on what went wrong, what you learned, and what you'll do differently next time. That's growth. When you start viewing life's struggles as training sessions for your mind, just like lifting weights for your body, you build emotional strength. Over time, you become calmer under pressure, more adaptable, and harder to knock down.

WHY TALKING IT OUT IS STRENGTH, NOT WEAKNESS

Here's the truth: no one can carry the load of life alone. At some point, we all need a sounding board: a friend, a mentor, a partner, a team member or a professional. Talking doesn't mean you've lost control. It means you care enough about yourself to do something before things spiral. It's the release valve that stops pressure from exploding.

Start small. Share how your week's been. Admit when something's weighing on you. Chances are that the person next to you has been through something similar. You'll be surprised how quickly vulnerability builds connection and how much lighter you feel when you stop carrying it alone.

Remember: courage isn't found in silence. It's found in honesty.

SMALL DAILY HABITS FOR MENTAL FITNESS

Emotional wellness isn't just about avoiding breakdowns, it's about building daily habits that keep your mind fit and flexible.

Here are a few to keep in your mental toolkit:

1. Gratitude check-in:

Each morning or evening, jot down three things you're grateful for. It sounds simple, but it rewires your brain to focus on what's working, not what's missing.

2. Move your body:

Exercise is one of the best mental health tools there is. It boosts mood, lowers anxiety, and clears your head. You're never more than one workout away from feeling better.

3. Breathe and pause:

Take 5 minutes a day to simply stop, breathe deeply, close your eyes, and slow things down. Your nervous system needs moments of calm to reset.

4. Connect:

Call a friend. Have a chat over coffee. Join a sporting team or a community group. Social connection is medicine, and it keeps you accountable. Connection must be more than a text, a voicemail or an email. It must be face-to-face, verbal, with eye contact.

5. Limit the noise:

Too much news, social media, or negativity drains your mental battery. Protect your attention like it's your most valuable resource, because it is.

6. Reflect, don't react:

Instead of exploding or retreating when life gets stressful, pause and reflect. Ask yourself, *'What's really going on here?'*. That small gap between reaction and response is where wisdom lives.

THE REAL STRENGTH LIES WITHIN YOU

The strongest person isn't the one who never falls, they are the one who keeps getting back up, learning, and moving forward. Emotional wellness isn't about being unshakable, it's about being aware. It's knowing when to rest, when to talk, and when to ask for help. When you take care of your inner world, your outer world transforms, your relationships deepen, your focus sharpens, and your purpose becomes clearer. So drop the mask. Be real. Be open. Because the toughest thing isn't to hide your emotions, it's to own them. Your physical strength gets you through the day. Your emotional strength gets you through life. The key to longevity is building both and protecting both.

TOP 3 TIPS TO IMPROVE EMOTIONAL WELLBEING

1. ACKNOWLEDGE YOUR FEELINGS

Emotional strength starts with awareness, not avoidance. Name what you feel; it will help you to process, release, and grow from it. Remember: you can't heal what you don't feel.

2. NURTURE MEANINGFUL CONNECTIONS

Spend time with people who lift you up and allow you to be real. Genuine conversations and shared laughter are powerful emotional medicine.

3. CREATE SPACE TO RESET

Prioritise quiet time (walk, journal, meditate, or simply breathe), as stillness allows your mind to declutter and your emotions to realign.

LIST THREE ACTIONABLE STEPS TO IMPROVE YOUR EMOTIONAL WELLBEING

1._____

2._____

3._____

CHAPTER 6

FRIENDSHIP AND SOCIAL CONNECTIVITY:
Don't Go It Alone

"No man is an island. No man stands alone."

~ John Donne

There's a silent epidemic affecting people across the world and it's not just about physical health. The epidemic is isolation. Too many people are doing life solo, quietly carrying the load, trying to 'handle it' on their own, but here's the truth: connection isn't a luxury, it's a lifeline. We're wired for community. From ancient tribes to modern teams, we have always thrived when surrounded by other people who've got you back. Yet in today's fast-paced, digital world, that sense of togetherness has slipped away, replaced by busyness, pride, and quiet disconnection. So, in this chapter, I want you to reclaim your social connectivity or help others to reclaim theirs. Remember, help one, help many.

THE POWER OF CONNECTION IN HEALTH OPTIMISATION

Strong social bonds aren't just good for the soul, they are good for your body too. Studies show that meaningful relationships lower stress, reduce the risk of depression, strengthen the immune system, and even extend lifespan. Connection gives people purpose, perspective, and a sense of belonging. When you're surrounded by good people, friends who listen, challenge, and support you, life feels lighter. You show up stronger at work, at home, and within yourself. Being part of a tribe isn't weakness, it is part of your DNA. It's your biology. It's how we are built to survive and thrive.

WHY ISOLATION IS TOXIC

The simple fact is, loneliness kills. It's been linked to higher rates of heart disease, addiction, anxiety, and suicide. Yet too often when the going gets tough, the first thing we do is isolate. We tell ourselves, "I don't want to be a burden," or "I'll sort it out myself." However, the longer we stay silent, the heavier the weight becomes, and isolation feeds on negative thinking. It turns molehills into mountains.

When you open up even just a little you break that toxic cycle, and give others permission to do the same. That's where healing begins. Become the leader and eliminate isolation. Why? Because a strong network of friends can be the difference between sinking and surviving. Whether it's a friend checking in with a simple, *"You good?"*, or someone dragging you out for a surf, a gym session, a shopping trip, a beer or a wine, those small moments matter. Connection gives perspective, and it reminds you that you're not alone, that everyone struggles, and that together, you can get through anything.

Real friendship isn't about surface-level banter, it's about trust. It's being there when it counts. Listening without judgment. Calling out the bullshit. Offering support when a friend is too proud to ask for it. The strongest relationships are with those who are there through thick and thin. They are willing to stand shoulder to shoulder with you regardless of circumstance.

Having worked in the health and wellness industry for over two decades, something powerful happens when you surround yourself with good people. You lift each other higher. You celebrate wins, share struggles, and keep each other on track.

That's what life is all about: having a team that challenges you to do better and be better. To train harder. Eat cleaner. Be more present. Live with purpose and passion. It's why teams, gyms, groups, and local communities matter. They create structure, belonging, and momentum. When you fall off the wagon and throughout your life and your wellness journey you will they are the ones who will pull you back on. I cannot stress enough the importance of having and creating a positive environment to thrive.

One of the key themes I talk a lot about in speaking engagements is 'the importance of establishing a TEAM. Why? Because people need stability, support and accountability. We all need a circle of people who support, challenge, and inspire us. The ones you can laugh with, lean on, and learn from.

Your TEAM might include:

- A best friend who keeps it real.

- A mentor who gives perspective.

- A training partner who pushes you harder.

- A work colleague who listens, no judgment.

- A community that makes you feel like you belong.

If you don't have that yet, then let's start to build it. Start by reaching out. The easiest way to do this is to say yes to that coffee, the walk, or the workout. The magic of connection doesn't happen by accident, it's built through small, consistent moments of showing up.

Remember: your environment shapes your energy. Surround yourself with people who make you better, not bitter. The lone wolf myth is dead. Strength isn't about doing everything yourself, it's about knowing when to lean in. You don't need hundreds of friends, you just need a handful of good ones who truly have your back. The ones who remind you who you are when life gets messy.

So, reach out. Reconnect. Be that person who checks in, listens, and leads by example, because when humans connect, we heal.

Throughout The Longevity Blueprint I talk a lot about The Perfect Threesome: Sleep, Nutrition and Exercise; but the foundation of health isn't isolated to these three dimensions alone. One of the key ingredients is connection, because when you've got a team behind you, you go further. You recover faster. You show up better. Connection keeps you grounded, accountable, and alive in every sense of the word.

TOP 3 TIPS TO IMPROVE SOCIAL CONNECTIVITY

1. BE PRESENT AND ENGAGED

Put the phone down, make eye contact, and truly listen. Genuine presence builds trust, deepens bonds, and reminds others they matter.

2. JOIN COMMUNITIES THAT SHARE YOUR VALUES

Surround yourself with people who inspire and support you. Whether it's a sports club, hobby group, or volunteering, connection grows through shared purpose and experiences.

3. REACH OUT REGULARLY

Don't wait for others to connect; take the first step. A simple message, coffee catch-up, or check-in call can make someone's day and strengthen your own sense of belonging.

LIST THREE ACTIONABLE STEPS TO IMPROVE YOUR CONNECTION

1._____

2._____

3._____

CHAPTER 7

HABITS, NOT HACKS:
The Real Secret to Lasting Change

"Success isn't built on motivation, it's built on habits. The small things you do daily become the big things that shape your life."

~ Tory Trewhitt

We live in a world obsessed with shortcuts: 6-week challenges, 30-day detoxes, miracle supplements, biohacking and quick-fix programs that promise the world and deliver a crash. But here's the uncomfortable truth: there are no shortcuts to sustainable health. You don't need hacks. You need habits. You have to do the basics before the biohacking. Real change doesn't happen overnight; it happens over time. It's not about intensity, it's about consistency. The person who trains three times a week for a year will always beat the person who goes all-out for a month every single time. This chapter is about building habits that stick; the kind that compound quietly and turn small wins into unstoppable momentum as you work your way to optimising your wellness.

One of the main reasons that I still get speaking gigs and work directly with humans as an accountability and health coach is simple: quick fixes feel exciting because they promise instant results and we love that dopamine hit, but motivation is temporary. When the hype fades and life gets busy, so do the results, and that is typically where I step in. The diet fails, the gym shoes gather dust, and the old habits return stronger than ever. That's because quick fixes target behaviour, not identity. They tell you what to do, not who to become. People say, 'Knowledge is Power', but I call BULLSHIT on this. IMPLEMENTATION is power! We all know what is right and wrong.

Think of it like this: if you see yourself as someone 'trying to get healthy', you'll always rely on willpower. However, when you start seeing yourself as a healthy person, your choices naturally align with that identity. You don't force it, you start living it.

Lasting change isn't about overhauling everything. It's about upgrading who you are, one small habit at a time.

Here's the golden rule: **start so small it's almost impossible to fail.**

Want to get fitter?
Start with 10 minutes of movement a day.
Want to eat better?
Add one serve of veggies to your dinner.
Want to sleep better?
Turn your phone off 15 minutes earlier.
The point isn't perfection, it's progress.

Once that small habit becomes automatic, you stack another one on top. That's called habit stacking:

the art of building powerful routines by linking new actions to existing ones. For example:

- After I brush my teeth, I'll stretch for two minutes.

- After my morning coffee, I'll write down one thing I'm grateful for.

- After I finish work, I'll go for a 15-minute walk before dinner.

Stacked over time, these micro-actions become the framework of a healthier, more disciplined life.

Many of my good mates are in the finance industry, trading their health for money. At some stage they will need to invest in themselves or risk spending all their money on their health. So don't become another corporate statistic; think of your habits like financial investments. A single deposit doesn't make you rich, but daily, consistent deposits compound into serious returns. The same goes for health. One workout won't transform you. One good night's sleep won't fix your energy. But do them regularly, and the results multiply. Consistency is the compound interest of success.

It's what separates those who 'try' from those who *become.*

Every time you follow through on a healthy choice, you reinforce your identity, and you cast a vote for the person you are becoming. Miss a day? No stress. Just don't miss two. Momentum loves consistency, not perfection.

Remember: the small things you do daily matter more than the big things you do occasionally. Habits require patience. You'll stumble. You'll skip days. You'll feel like nothing's changing. But keep showing up. Because one day, you'll wake up and realise the person who struggled to stay consistent *became* the person who doesn't know how to quit. That's the magic of habits. They turn effort into ease, and discipline into identity.

MASTER THE BORING STUFF

Anyone can get fired up for a new challenge. Few can master the mundane, the early alarms, the water bottle, the training sessions, the prep, the journaling, the check-ins. However, that's where greatness lives. In the repetition. In the quiet consistency no one sees. So, forget the hacks. Build habits. Stack them slowly. Protect them fiercely, because in the end, the person you become is simply the sum of what you do repeatedly.

TOP 3 TIPS TO IMPROVE YOUR HABITS

1. START SMALL, STAY CONSISTENT

Big change begins with small, repeatable actions. Focus on one habit at a time and make it so easy you can't fail. Consistency beats intensity every time.

2. LINK NEW HABITS TO EXISTING ONES

Use habit stacking: attach a new action to something you already do. Example: After brushing your teeth → stretch for 2 minutes. It's structure, not willpower, that drives success.

3. TRACK, REFLECT, AND REWARD

Measure your progress to build momentum and motivation. Celebrate small wins and learn from slip-ups. Remember: habits grow through awareness, not perfection.

LIST THREE ACTIONABLE STEPS TO IMPROVE YOUR DAILY HABITS

1._____

2._____

3._____

CHAPTER 8

THE BLUEPRINT:
Creating Your Longevity Formula

"Longevity isn't about living forever: it's about living well. Every choice you make today is an investment in the energy, strength, and clarity you'll have tomorrow."

~Tory Trewhitt

I f you've made it this far, you've probably realised something powerful: this isn't just about health, it's about ownership. It's about deciding that life isn't something that happens to you, but something you actively shape. By getting this far in the book, you have built awareness around your sleep, sharpened your focus on nutrition, learned the discipline of movement, found tools to tame stress, faced the weight of emotional health, rediscovered the strength in friendships and committed to building habits that last. Together, these aren't just lifestyle pillars; they're the foundations of a bigger game.

In my first book, BLOKES INC. I used 'Playing a Bigger Game' as a tag line, meaning taking ownership of the lifestyle you'd like to live. It's not about being perfect, it's about being intentional. Every decision, every rep, every conversation becomes part of the story you're writing about who you are. Unfortunately, too many people drift through life reacting to things, work stress, relationships, routines without ever asking, *"Is this the life I want?"*

Playing a Bigger Game means flipping that script. It means leading your own life instead of being led by circumstance. Stop chasing short-term pleasure and start investing in long-term fulfillment. Stop competing with others and start striving to outdo the person you were yesterday. It doesn't matter how much money you earn, how many hours you work, or how many responsibilities you juggle: if your health fails, everything else crumbles. However, when you prioritise your wellness, your sleep, your food, your movement and your mindset, every other part of life improves. You think clearer. You perform better. You show up stronger for the people who matter most. You realise that being healthy isn't selfish, it's strategic, because when you take care of yourself, you can take care of everyone else far more effectively.

There is no doubt that during your wellness journey you will stumble, you will slip back into old habits, you will lose motivation. That's all part of the process.

The difference between those who change and those who don't isn't failure, it's response. Do you beat yourself up and quit? Or do you reflect, recalibrate, and get back on track? Every setback is feedback. Every failure teaches you something that success can't. The bigger game isn't about avoiding failure, it's about playing through it.

TOP 3 TIPS TO START YOUR LONGEVITY JOURNEY

1. NOURISH YOUR BODY WITH REAL FOOD

Focus on whole, colourful, nutrient-dense foods. Eat mostly plants, include quality protein, and stay hydrated. What you eat today shapes how you age tomorrow.

2. MOVE DAILY WITH PURPOSE AND JOY

Walk, swim, lift, stretch — just keep moving. Regular, moderate activity boosts heart health, mobility, and mood. Longevity thrives on consistency, not intensity.

3. PRIORITISE REST AND RECOVERY

Sleep is your body's natural repair system. Aim for 7 — 9 hours and maintain a regular bedtime routine. Restoration fuels resilience and long-term vitality.

LIST THREE ACTIONABLE STEPS TO IMPROVE YOUR LONGEVITY JOURNEY

1._____

2._____

3._____

CHAPTER 9

THE LEGACY YOU LEAVE

One day, your kids, your friends, or the people you lead will look at how you lived, not what you said. Did you model health? Did you chase purpose? Did you live with gratitude, energy, and intention? That's your legacy.

Not the trophies, not the titles, not your bank balance, but the way you showed up.

The Perfect Threesome is all about doing the basics well. Focusing on the 80/20 rule. Being honest and leading by example, taking responsibility, addressing what needs to be changed, staying consistent, seeking help if and when required and living life with courage and conviction.

You don't need to overhaul everything today. The Longevity Blueprint will give you the structure to do this, you just need to start by making one good choice at a time.

- Get to bed 30 minutes earlier.

- Add real food to your plate.

- Go for that walk.

- Call your friend.

- Take a breath before reacting.

Do the small things well, repeatedly, and watch your world expand, because the bigger game isn't 'out there', it's being played right here, right now, in the way you live today.

The world doesn't need more people chasing hustle. Instagramming their day-to-day activities, posting on Facebook or TikTok. The world needs more people chasing health, meaning, and connection. I encourage you to be that person. The person who has that strength, who isn't just focused on your job title, the car you drive, the suburb you live in, the holidays you have or the amount of money you earn. You understand that, The Perfect Threesome is really about honesty, accountability, discipline and purpose, first and foremost.

Be that person who sets the tone. Be the person who *Plays a Bigger Game.*

Your time is now.

Much love,

Tory

PERSONAL LONGEVITY CONTRACT

This contract is my commitment to myself, to live with intention, discipline, and purpose. By signing below, I acknowledge that my health, mindset, relationship and daily choices shape the quality of my life. This is my promise to build and follow the Longevity Blueprint.

MY COMMITMENTS

1. **I Commit to My Health -** I will prioritise movement, nutrition, sleep and recovery because my body is my foundation. I understand that longevity is not luck, it's consistency.

   MyPledge:_____

   _____

2. **I Commit to My Mindset -** I will cultivate resilience, gratitude and self awareness. I will choose growth over comfort and action over excuses.

   MyPledge:_____

   _____

3. **I Commit to My Relationships -** I will build strong connections, communicate clearly, and show up for the people who matter. I understand that real longevity included emotional and social wellbeing,

   MyPledge:_____

   _____

4. I Commit to Purposeful Action - I will take responsibility for my habits and behaviours. I will hold myself accountable to the human I want to become.

My Pledge:_____

_____

MY LONGEVITY BLUEPRINT

By signing this contract, I commit to living proactively, not reactively and to build a life aligned with my highest potential.

Three actions I will implement immediately;

1.

2.

3.

Signature

Name_____

Date_____

Signature_____

www.ingramcontent.com/pod-product-compliance
Lightning Source LLC
Chambersburg PA
CBHW060256030426
42335CB00014B/1729